FEMININE SEXUALITY:

WHAT EVERY WOMAN SHOULD KNOW ABOUT HER SEXUAL LIFE

BY

STEPHANIE W. CROOKS

TABLE OF CONTENTS

INTRODUCTION

A female of a particular age cannot become pregnant. Both the boy and the girl are unable to reproduce at an approximate age range. Because the boy's spermatozoa are not yet formed at this age, he will not be able to impregnate the female during this time. The female, on the other hand, has not yet begun to produce the eggs that would accept the male's sperm deposit. Thus, pregnancy is not possible.

CHAPTER 1

PUBERTY

The process by which a child's body develops into an adult body capable of sexual reproduction is known as puberty. It is started by hormonal impulses that travel from the brain to the gonads, which in a boy are the testicles, and the ovaries in a girl. The gonads create hormones in response to the signals, which promote libido as well as the development of the brain, bones, muscles, blood, skin, hair, breasts, and sex organs. Puberty typically affects both sexes, albeit the timing of some puberty symptoms varies depending on gender.

SIGNS OF PUBERTY IN GIRLS

Breast Development

The earliest physical symptom of puberty in girls is typically a firm, sensitive lump under the center of one or both breasts, which appears on average at around 10.5 years old. Thelarche is the name for this. This is stage 2 of breast development according to the commonly used Tanner staging of puberty (stage 1 is a flat, prepubertal breast). Within 6–12 months, the swelling had manifestly started on both sides, eased, and could be felt and seen expanding beyond the boundaries of the areolae. The third stage of breast development is at this point. By another 12 months (stage 4), the breasts will be nearing their mature size and shape, with the areolae and nipples forming a secondary mound. Although there is so much variance in the sizes and shapes of adult breasts that stage 4 and 5 are not often clearly distinguishable, in the majority of young women, this mound fades into the contour of the mature breast (stage 5).

Pubic Hairs

Usually occurring a few months after thelarche, pubic hair is frequently the second distinct change during puberty. Pubarche is the term used to describe it. Along the labia, the pubic hairs are typically the first to be noticed. Tanner stage 2 is used to describe the initial few hairs. Stage 3 is typically achieved in another 6 to 12 months at which point the pubic mound also develops too many hairs to count. By stage 4, the "pubic triangle" is firmly covered in pubic hair. Stage 5 describes the extension of pubic hair to the thighs and, on occasion, the upward growth of abdominal hair towards the navel. The first pubic hair begins to grow in 15% of girls before breast growth does.

Vagina, Uterus, Ovaries

Estrogen's action on the perineal skin causes it to keratinize, boosting its infection resistance. Increasing estrogen levels also cause changes to the mucosal surface of the vagina, which thickens and loses some of its pink tints (in contrast to the brighter red of the prepubertal vaginal mucosa). With a top layer of squamous cells, the mucosa develops into a multilayered structure. Glycogen content in the vaginal epithelium increases as a result of estrogen use, and this eventually plays a significant role in preserving the pH of the vagina. A typical estrogen consequence is the production of white discharges (physiologic leukorrhea). The size of the uterus, ovaries, and ovarian follicles all rise in the two years following thelarche. Small follicular cysts can typically be seen on ultrasound images of the ovaries. The uterine body-to-cervix ratio is 1:1 before pubertal development; it rises to 2:1 or 3:1 following the pubertal phase.

Menstruation and Fertility

Menarche is the term used to describe the onset of the first menstrual period, which normally happens two years after thelarche. In the US, 12.5 is the average age of menarche. The majority of American females start their periods between the ages of 11 and 12 or 13, however, some start after turning 14 and some before turning 11. In actuality, a range of 8 to 16 is considered normal. Menarche typically occurs at 12.72 years of age in Canada and 12.9 years in the UK. In the first two years following menarche, the intervals between menses are not usually regular. The early menses may or may not be accompanied by ovulation, which is crucial for fertility. About 80% of the cycles in postmenarchal girls were anovulatory in the first year following menarche, 50% in the third year, and 10% in the sixth year. It's not always the case that ovulation will begin following menarche. Many females who experience persistent irregularity in their menstrual cycle several years after menarche will continue to experience extended irregularity and anovulation, and they are more likely to experience decreased fertility.

The lower portion of the pelvis and consequently the hips broaden during this time due to growing estrogen levels (providing a larger birth canal). Particularly in the usual feminine distribution of breasts, hips, buttocks, thighs, upper arms, and pubis, fat tissue rises to a bigger percentage of the body composition than in males. By the end of adolescence, the typical female body shape is a result of progressive variances in fat distribution as well as sex differences in local skeletal growth. Girls have 6% more body fat than boys do on average when they are 10 years old.

Acne and body odor

Rising androgen levels can alter the fatty acid makeup of sweat, giving off a more "adult"-smelling body odor. This frequently occurs one or more years before thelarche and pubarche. Sebum production from the skin increases, which is another impact of androgens. This alteration makes people more vulnerable to acne, a skin disorder linked to puberty. The severity of acne varies widely.

Visual and other impacts of hormonal changes

The main female sex hormone, estradiol, thickens the lips and oral mucosa in girls and promotes the growth of the vulva. Estradiol causes the myoepithelial layer and smooth muscle of the vagina to develop as well as the skin to thicken (stratify) in the vulva and vagina. Estradiol typically causes the labia majora to develop less noticeably and the labia minora to grow more noticeably. Estradiol is also responsible for the increased pheomelanin production that gives the lips, labia minora, and occasionally labia majora their distinctive red color. The deeper pigmentation of the areola is also brought on by estradiol and other ovarian steroids.

The clitoris will enlarge due to testosterone, and it may also have significant effects on the maturation and expansion of the vestibular bulbs, clitoris corpus cavernosum, and urethral sponge.

The lower urinary tract appears to be impacted by changes to the vulva that estradiol causes as well as its direct effects.

Armpit hair

Under the arms, new hair grows, initially scant before becoming thicker and darker with time.

SIGNS OF PUBERTY IN BOYS

The growth of the testicles and scrotum marks the start of puberty in boys. In addition, the penis grows larger, and a boy grows pubic hair. Sperm production also starts in a boy's testicles. Ejaculation is the act of releasing semen, which contains sperm and other fluids. When a boy reaches puberty, his erect penis develops the ability to ejaculate semen and impregnate a female. A boy's first ejaculation is a significant developmental turning point. A kid typically has his first ejaculation at age 13. Nocturnal emission is the term for ejaculation that occasionally happens while a person is sleeping.

Testicular size

The first outward sign of puberty in boys is the growth of the testicles (and is termed gonadarche). From the time a boy reaches about the age of one until the beginning of puberty, the size of his testicles remains relatively constant, averaging about 2-3 cm in length and about 1.5-2 cm in width. The Tanner scale for male genitalia has parameters that range from stage I, which indicates a volume of less than 1.5 ml, to stage V, which represents a testicular volume of larger than 20 ml. One of these criteria is the size of the testicles. Six years following the commencement of puberty, testicular growth achieves its maximum adult size. While the average adult testicular volume is 18 to 20 cm3, the typical population's testicular sizes vary greatly. The length and then the breadth of the penis' shaft will grow, and the glans penis and corpora cavernosa will also start to enlarge to adult dimensions after the boy's testicles have enlarged and developed for about a year.

Male body type and musculature

Adult men have denser bones and almost twice as much skeletal muscle by the time puberty is over. Male and female skeletal forms differ substantially as a result of some of the bone growth, which is disproportionately bigger in some areas (such as shoulder breadth and jaw). The average adult male has around 50% more body fat and roughly 150% more lean body mass than the average adult female. This muscle grows mostly in the latter stages of puberty, and it can continue to grow even after a male has reached biological adulthood. About a year after

a male reaches his peak growth rate, the so-called "strength surge," or rate of muscular growth, reaches its peak.
Male nipples and fat pads of male breast tissue frequently form during adolescence; occasionally, particularly in one breast, this becomes more obvious and is known as gynecomastia. Typically, it is a transient event.

Erections
Medically referred to as nocturnal penile tumescence and colloquially known as morning wood, erections occur while sleeping or when you first get up. The penis can frequently become erected while a person is sleeping, and men or boys frequently awaken with an erection. Puberty causes erections to happen substantially more frequently in teenage boys. Erections can happen on their own at any time of the day, and if you're wearing clothes, they might leave a bulge or "hump." Wearing tight-fitting undergarments, a long shirt, and baggier clothing can help to conceal or mask this. Male infants and prepubescent youngsters frequently experience erections, and this can even happen before the baby is even born. Spontaneous erections usually referred to as unwanted or involuntary

erections, are common.

Retraction of the foreskin

A boy's foreskin widens during puberty, if not earlier, and eventually should allow for painless retraction down the penis shaft and behind the glans. The membrane that connects the inner surface of the foreskin to the glans separates, allowing the foreskin to stand alone from the glans. The foreskin then gradually begins to retract. According to research by Oster (1968), as puberty progressed, more boys were able to pull back their foreskins. At ages 12 to 13, they discovered that only 60% of boys could retract their foreskins; by ages 14 to 15, this number rose to 85%; and at ages 16 to 17, it reached 95%. He also discovered that, between the ages of 14 and 17, 1% of individuals who were unable to retract had phimosis, while the other 93% were only partially able to do so. Ishikawa and Kawakita (2004) discovered that by the age of 15, 77% of their sample of boys could retract their foreskins, supporting the findings of earlier research by Kayaba et al. (1996) on a sample of over 600 boys. Boys may benefit from manual stretching in Beaugé's (1997) report to help the development of retractile foreskin.

Penile hygiene should be an integral part of a boy's daily self-care regimen after he can retract his foreskin. Numerous studies recommend that boys be taught the importance of hygiene, including retracting the foreskin while urinating and rinsing under it and around the glans at each opportunity to bathe, despite the American Academy of Pediatrics statement that there is "little evidence to affirm the association between circumcision status and optimal penile hygiene." Krueger and Osborn (1986) discovered that routine washing under the foreskin lowers the incidence of a variety of penile problems; nevertheless, Birley et al. (1993) suggest that excessive washing with soap should be avoided since it dries the tissues' oils and can result in non-specific dermatitis.

Pubic hair

Boys frequently develop pubic hair immediately after their genitalia start to expand. The dorsal (abdominal) root of the penis is typically where the pubic hairs are first discernible. Stage 2 is referred to as the first few hairs. Stage 3 is often attained in another 6 to 12 months when there are too many hairs to count. By stage 4, the "pubic triangle" is firmly covered in pubic hair. Stage 5 describes the spread of pubic hair to the thighs and up toward the navel as a component of the developing abdominal hair.

Hair on the body and the face

Other skin regions that react to androgens may also grow androgenic hair in the months and years after pubic hair first appears. Underarm (axillary) hair, perianal hair, upper lip hair, sideburn (preauricular) hair, periareolar hair, and the beard region are the typical order of growth. This particular order may differ for certain people, as it does for the majority of biological processes in humans. Hair on the arms, legs, chest, abdomen, and back gets heavier more gradually. Adult men have a wide range of body hair amounts, and there are notable variations in the time and amount of hair growth among various racial groups. In late adolescence, facial hair is frequently present, however, it may not start to grow until much later. After puberty, facial hair will continue to grow thicker, darker, and coarser for an additional two to four years. Some males don't start growing full facial hair until up to 10 years after adolescence is over. Although not all men get chest hair, it might start to sprout during adolescence or years afterward.

Adam's apple and voice changes

Both sexes experience growth of the larynx (or voice box) when androgens are present. The male voice drops and deepens, occasionally abruptly but seldom "overnight," by around one octave, as a result of this maturation, which is much more pronounced in boys since their longer and thicker vocal folds have a lower fundamental frequency. The larynx of both males and girls is around the same size before puberty. In the beginning stages of untrained voices, a voice change can occasionally be accompanied by unsteadiness of vocalization. During stages 3–4 of male puberty, at around the time of peak growth, the majority of the voice change occurs. Adult pitch is acquired at an average age of 15 years, although the voice may not entirely settle until the early twenties. It frequently precedes the development of considerable facial hair for several months to years.

CHAPTER 2
VARIATIONS

Reproductive maturity marks the end of puberty, generally speaking. The accomplishment of the ability to reproduce, the attainment of the maximum adult height, the maximum gonadal size, or the levels of adult sex hormones are among the criteria that may be used to define the conclusion for various purposes. A typical girl reaches her maximum adult height at the age of 15, whereas a typical boy does so at the age of 18. Potential fertility, also known as nubility, typically occurs 1-2 years before growth is finished in girls and 3-4 years before growth is finished in boys. Stage 5 often denotes the peak of adult hormone production and gonadal development.

The starting age

The criteria for when puberty begins may vary depending on the viewpoint (e.g., hormonal versus physical) and the goal (establishing population normal standards, clinical care of early or late pubescent individuals, etc.). Physical alterations to a person's body are a typical characterization of the start of puberty. These bodily alterations are the initial outward manifestations of altered neuronal, hormonal, and gonadal activity.

The onset of puberty varies from person to person; typically, it happens between the ages of 10 and 13. Both genetic and environmental factors, such as nutrition status and social situations, have an impact on the age at which puberty starts. The Vandenbergh effect is an illustration of social circumstances; it states that young girls who contact adult males frequently before they reach puberty do so earlier than young girls who do not.

Race may also have an impact on the typical age of puberty. For instance, the average age of menarche has been shown to range from 12 to 18 years throughout the populations studied. African-American females experience the earliest average beginning of puberty, while high-altitude subsistence tribes in Asia experience the later average onset. However, a significant shift in food within a few generations can significantly alter many of the higher age averages, which more often than not reflect nutritional restrictions than genetic variations. A population's median age at menarche may serve as a proxy for the number of malnourished girls in that population, and a population's distribution of wealth and food may be reflected in the width of the spread.

Researchers have found that puberty can start sooner than previously thought. The comparison of data from 1999 with data from 1969, however, served as the foundation for their conclusions. A small sample of white girls served as the sample population in the preceding case (200, from Britain). According to later research, 48% of African-American girls and 12% of white girls by the age of nine experience puberty.

Kallmann syndrome, a type of hypogonadotropic hypogonadism, is one potential factor that could contribute to a delay in the onset of puberty past the ages of 14 for girls and 15 for boys (HH). Lack of smell is another symptom of Kallmann disease (anosmia). Both men and women can get HH, including Kallmann syndrome. It is brought on by a breakdown in the HPG axis at puberty, which leads to low or absent gonadotropin (LH and FSH) levels, which have the knock-on effects of puberty not starting or finishing, secondary hypogonadism, and infertility.

Since the 1840s, the average age at which puberty begins has decreased dramatically. The average age of menarche among Western European females decreased by four months in each of the ten years from 1840 to 1950. Girls born in Norway in 1840 typically reached menarche at the age of 17. 15.3 years was the national average in France in 1840. The average age in England in 1840 was 16.5

years. In Japan, the fall occurred later and then more quickly: there was an 11-month decline there every ten years from 1945 to 1975.

According to a 2006 Danish study, puberty began at an average age of 9 years and 10 months, one year earlier than when a related study was conducted in 1991. The phenomenon, which increases girls' long-term risk of breast cancer, may be related to obesity or exposure to toxins in the food chain, according to scientists.

Environmental influences and Genetic determinants
In well-nourished communities, the timing of puberty varies by at least 46% due to direct genetic factors, according to numerous studies. The genetic correlation between timing and mothers and daughters is the highest. The precise genes that control time are still unknown. An androgen receptor gene is one of the contenders. Researchers have proposed that certain hair care products that include estrogen or placenta, as well as certain chemicals, specifically phthalates, which are present in many cosmetics, toys, and plastic food containers, may contribute to the early beginning of puberty. Given that hereditary variables only explain 50% of the diversity in pubertal timing, environmental factors must also play a

significant role. Puberty takes longer to develop in children raised at higher elevations, which is one of the first environmental consequences to be noticed. Although nutrition is undoubtedly the most significant environmental factor, other factors have also been discovered that have a greater impact on the timing of female puberty and menarche than male puberty.

Steroids and hormones

Environmental hormones and chemicals may have an impact on human prenatal or postnatal sexual development, according to theory and animal research. Large quantities of estrogens and progestogens from pharmaceutical items are discharged into the sewage systems of big cities and are occasionally found in the environment. Although they are occasionally utilized in cattle farming, sex steroids are no longer permitted in the production of chicken meat. Although agricultural laws control uses to reduce unintentional human intake, the laws are mostly self-enforced in the United States. Some or all of the changes associated with puberty may be brought on by a child being exposed to hormones or other substances that activate the estrogen or androgen receptors.

Environmental pollutants like PCBs (polychlorinated biphenyls), which can bind to and activate estrogen receptors, are more widely dispersed and therefore more difficult to identify as influences on puberty.

When young children are evaluated medically for premature puberty, more pronounced degrees of partial puberty caused by direct exposure to modest but considerable amounts of pharmaceutical sex steroids at home may be found, but moderate effects and the other probable exposures mentioned above would not.

Plastics are produced using the chemical bisphenol A (BPA), which is widely found in infant bottles, water bottles, sporting goods, medical equipment, and cans of food and beverages. Due to its potential to disrupt the mammary gland, and the prostate gland, and promote early puberty in females, scientists are worried about the behavioral consequences of BPA on fetuses, newborns, and children at current exposure levels. Estrogen, a key regulator of development and reproduction, is imitated by BPA, which disrupts its activity. The Centers for Disease Control and Prevention (CDC) identified detectable levels of BPA in the bodies of more than 90% of the U.S. population examined. BPA seeps out of the plastic into beverages and foods. Children and babies are thought to consume the most BPA regularly.

BPA is present in many plastic baby bottles, and when plastic is heated, such as when warming a baby bottle or warming food in the microwave, BPA is more likely to leach out of the material.

Dietary influence

The environmental elements that have the greatest and most direct impact on when puberty occurs are nutritional ones. Because they must provide all of the nutrition for a developing baby, girls are particularly sensitive to nutritional management. Body fat percentage reflects excess calories (calories consumed more than needed for growth and exercise), which tells the brain there are enough calories to start puberty and have children. Numerous pieces of evidence indicate that over most of the last few centuries, dietary variations were largely responsible for the diversity in pubertal timing among populations and even within social classes within the same society. Puberty ages have recently decreased, especially in populations with higher prior ages, as a result of recent worldwide increases in the consumption of animal protein, other changes in diet, and increases in childhood obesity. The amount of variation that can be attributed to nutrition is decreasing in many populations. Although the most significant dietary influence on the timing of puberty is available dietary energy (simple calories), food quality also matters. Female puberty starts later and advances more slowly when there are lower protein intakes and higher dietary fiber intakes, which are typical of vegetarian diets.

Influence of obesity and Exercise

Early obesity and the start of puberty in girls have been connected by scientists. Breast development before the age of nine and menarche before the age of twelve have been linked to fat. Girls' early puberty may be a sign of future health issues.

It has also been demonstrated that physical activity levels, particularly in females, have an impact on the timing of puberty. High levels of exercise lower the energy calories available for reproduction and delay puberty, whether it is done for athletic, body-image, or daily survival reasons. A decreased body fat mass and cholesterol frequently enhance the effects of exercise.

Mental and Physical Illness

Both boys and girls can postpone puberty due to chronic illnesses. The ones that involve persistent inflammation or interfere with nutrition have the biggest impact. In the past century, TB and inflammatory bowel disease have become known in the west for having such an impact, although persistent parasitic infections are common in poor regions of the world.

Puberty is when mental diseases first appear. Hormones play a key role in the development of the brain, which can affect mood disorders such as schizophrenia, bipolar disorder, major depressive disorder, and dysthymia. 40% of anorexia nervosa cases between the ages of 15 and 19 involve females.

Social influences and stress

Social and psychological factors are some of the least understood environmental impacts on when puberty occurs. Social variables have a limited impact on timing, altering it by a few months rather than years compared to the effects of genetics, nutrition, and general health. The underlying physiological mechanisms of these social impacts, including pheromones, have been the subject of numerous hypotheses based on animal studies, although they are not yet fully understood.

The family is the most significant component of a child's psychosocial environment, and the majority of social impact research has examined aspects of family structure and function in connection with earlier or later female puberty.

The majority of studies have found that girls living in high-stress environments, whose fathers are absent during their early years, who have a stepfather in the house, who experience prolonged sexual abuse as children, or who are adopted from a developing country at a young age may experience menarche a few months earlier. When a girl grows up in a big family with her biological father, menarche might happen a little later than usual.

The delay of maturation has been linked to more severe levels of environmental stress, such as being a refugee during a war with a threat to one's physical existence; this effect may be exacerbated by inadequacy in one's food. Most of these social consequences that have been recorded are minor, and our knowledge of them is lacking.

The majority of these "effects" are statistical relationships discovered through epidemiological studies. There are many covariables and possible alternative explanations; statistical relationships are not always causal. Effects on a child of such a little size cannot be proven or disproven. The ease with which this type of study can be exploited for political advocacy makes interpretations of the data politically contentious as well. Sometimes, criticism of science is accompanied by allegations of prejudice based on political agenda.

Another drawback of social research is that almost all of it has focused on females. This is because female puberty demands more physiological resources and also because it entails a special event (menarche), which makes survey research on female puberty much easier than male puberty.

Sequence variations

There are times when the order of events during pubertal development can change. For instance, in 15% of boys and girls, pubarche (the first pubic hairs) may occur many months before gonadarche and thelarche, respectively. Rarely, menarche can start before other indicators of puberty in some girls. These variations need to be examined by a doctor because they occasionally signify a sickness.

CHAPTER 3
DEVELOPMENT OF PREGNANCY

Pregnancy is the period when one or more offspring (gestates) develop inside a woman's uterus (womb). The time of growth during which viviparous animals carry an embryo, and eventually a fetus, is known as gestation (the embryo develops within the parent). It frequently occurs in mammals but also in some non-mammals. During pregnancy, mammals may have one or more gestations concurrently, as in the case of multiple births.

The gestation period is the period throughout gestation. Gestational age, which is usually equal to the age of conception + two weeks, is the time since the first menstrual period, in the field of obstetrics.
Clinical or biochemical criteria can be used to define pregnancy in humans. According to medical standards, pregnancy begins the day after the mother's last period. Pregnancy begins biochemically when a woman's human

chorionic gonadotropin (hCG) levels exceed 25 mIU/mL. The first, second, and third trimesters of human pregnancy are each roughly three months long and are referred to as trimesters. The first trimester lasts from the end of the last period until the thirteenth week, the second trimester lasts from the fourteenth week through the twenty-eighth and nineteenth weeks, and the third trimester lasts from the twenty-ninth and nineteenth weeks to the forty-second week. The gestational age at which birth often occurs is around 40 weeks, although births can also happen between 37 and 42 weeks. Preterm labor, which occurs before 37 weeks of pregnancy, can be caused by several things, including previous preterm births.

Prenatal care is crucial for the upkeep of a healthy pregnancy and the monitoring of associated issues. Prenatal care in high-income nations typically consists of monthly visits for the first two trimesters, increasing in frequency as the due date approaches. During these appointments, medical professionals will assess a range of parental and fetal metrics, including the growth and heart rate of the fetus, birth abnormalities, and the mother's blood pressure, among others.

To estimate the gestational age, medical professionals will weigh the newborn, and assess their vital signs, reflexes, head circumference, muscle tone, and posture. Pregnancy-related illnesses and receiving sufficient prenatal care are just two factors that can affect how long a pregnancy lasts. In the United States, the prevalence of morbidity and pre-existing conditions that put mothers at risk for potentially fatal pregnancy-related complications is rising. Non-Hispanic Black women bear the bulk of this load. This persistent difference could be partially explained by the lack of accessibility to prenatal care. Socioeconomic position, insurance status, daycare, social support, housing, and immigration status are other variables that influence the use of prenatal care.

CHAPTER 4

MISCARRIAGE

A miscarriage is the death of an embryo or fetus before it can survive on its own. It is also referred to medically as a spontaneous abortion and pregnancy loss. ESHRE classifies miscarriage before six weeks of gestation as a biochemical loss. Clinical miscarriage, which can occur early before 12 weeks and late between 12 and 21 weeks, is the term used once ultrasound or histology evidence demonstrates that pregnancy has existed. A stillbirth occurs when a fetus dies after 20 weeks of gestation. Vaginal bleeding with or without discomfort is the most typical miscarriage symptom. Afterward, it's possible to feel sad, anxious, or guilty. Tissue and clot-like material can travel through and out of the vagina after leaving the uterus. Recurrent miscarriages, sometimes known as RSAs or recurrent spontaneous abortions, are also sometimes seen as a type of infertility.

Older parents, past miscarriages, exposure to tobacco smoke, obesity, diabetes, thyroid issues, and drug or alcohol usage are risk factors for miscarriage. Within the first 12 weeks of pregnancy, miscarriages account for about 80% of cases (the first trimester). Chromosomal abnormalities are the underlying cause in roughly 50% of instances. The cervix's state, hCG blood levels, and an ultrasound may all be used to diagnose a miscarriage. Similar symptoms can also be caused by an ectopic pregnancy and implantation hemorrhage.

In some cases, prevention is achievable with quality prenatal care. The chance of miscarriage may be reduced by avoiding drugs, alcohol, infectious disorders, radiation, and other factors. Typically, no special care is required in the first 7 to 14 days. Most miscarriages end on their own without further treatment. The leftover tissue is occasionally removed with the drug misoprostol or a method like a vacuum aspiration. Rho(D) immune globulin may be necessary for women with rhesus-negative (Rh-negative) blood types. Painkillers might be useful. Processing the loss may be aided by emotional support.

The most frequent early pregnancy issue is miscarriage. Miscarriage rates among women who are aware of their pregnancy range from 10% to 20%, whereas rates throughout all fertilization range from 30% to 50%. The risk is approximately 10% in those under the age of 35 and approximately 45% in people over the age of 40. The age at which risk starts to rise is around 30. Two consecutive miscarriages occur in about 5% of women. To lessen distress, some advice not to use the word "abortion" in conversations with people who are having a miscarriage. The term "miscarriage" has taken the place of the phrase "spontaneous abortion" in Britain when referring to pregnancy loss and in response to accusations of being insensitive to those who had experienced such loss. This adjustment also helps to clear up any misunderstandings among non-medical professionals who might not be aware that "spontaneous abortion" refers to a naturally occurring medical occurrence rather than the deliberate termination of a pregnancy.

SIGNS AND SYMPTOMS OF MISCARRIAGE

Vaginal spotting, cramping, abdominal pain, and the passage of fluid, blood clots, and tissue from the vagina are all indications of a miscarriage. Although bleeding can be a sign of miscarriage, many people have bleeding in the first trimester of pregnancy without miscarrying. One term for bleeding during the first half of pregnancy is "threatened miscarriage." About half of the pregnant women who seek medical attention for bleeding will miscarry. During an ultrasound examination or through repeated human chorionic gonadotropin (HCG) tests, miscarriage may be identified.

RISK ELEMENTS FOR MISCARRIAGE

Miscarriage can happen for a variety of causes, not all of which are known. Risk factors are those variables that, while not always causing a miscarriage, enhance the chance of having one. Miscarriage risk is heightened by up to 70 diseases, infections, treatments, lifestyle choices, occupational exposures, chemical exposures, and shift employment. Endocrine, genetic, uterine, hormonal, and reproductive tract infections are a few of these dangers, along with tissue rejection brought on by an autoimmune condition.

TRIMESTERS

First trimester

According to several studies, the first trimester is when the majority of clinically evident miscarriages (between two-thirds and three-quarters) take place. About 30% to 40% of all fertilized eggs miscarry, frequently before the pregnancy is detected. Normally, the pregnancy is discharged before the embryo dies; but, in some cases, bleeding into the decidua basalis and tissue necrosis trigger uterine contractions to release the pregnancy. A placental or other embryonic tissue defects can cause early miscarriages. Sometimes, different tissues form instead of an embryo. This has been referred to as a "blighted ovum."

The zygote will most likely successfully implant into the uterus eight to ten days following fertilization. The likelihood of implantation decreases over the course of the next days if the zygote has not been implanted by day ten.

A chemical pregnancy is one that was discovered through testing but ends in miscarriage before or close to the start of the following anticipated period.

More than half of embryos lost during the first 13 weeks of pregnancy have chromosomal abnormalities. Aneuploidy accounts for 25% of all miscarriages or the loss of half of the embryo (abnormal number of chromosomes). Tetraploidy (2-4%), triploidy (6-8%), monosomy X (5-20%), autosomal trisomy (22-32%), or other structural chromosomal abnormalities (2%), are frequently detected in miscarriages. The increased rates seen in older women may be due to the higher likelihood of genetic issues with older parents.

Lack of progesterone during the luteal phase may or may not be a cause of miscarriage.

Second and Third trimesters

Losses in the second trimester may be brought on by maternal conditions such as uterine deformity, uterine growths (fibroids), or cervical issues. Premature birth may also be influenced by these diseases. Second-trimester miscarriages are less likely than first-trimester miscarriages to be brought on by a genetic disorder; chromosomal abnormalities are discovered in one-third of instances. A third-trimester infection may result in a miscarriage.

Age

A major risk factor is the pregnant woman's age. Age-related increases in the miscarriage rate are particularly pronounced after age 35. The risk is approximately 10% in those under the age of 35 and approximately 45% in people over the age of 40. The age at which risk starts to rise is around 30. The age of the father is linked to higher risk.

Caffeine, eating disorders, and obesity

Obesity is linked not only to miscarriage but also to subfertility and other unfavorable pregnancy outcomes. Obesity and recurrent miscarriage are connected. A higher risk of miscarriage may exist in women who suffer from anorexia nervosa or bulimia nervosa. Hyperemesis gravidarum can occasionally occur before a miscarriage, however, nutrient shortages have not been observed to affect miscarriage rates.

At least at higher ingestion levels, caffeine has also been linked to a greater likelihood of miscarriage. These higher rates, nevertheless, are only statistically significant under specific conditions.

The prevention of miscarriage has generally not been demonstrated to be aided by vitamin supplementation. There is no evidence that Chinese herbal medication can stop miscarriages.

Endocrine issues

Pregnancy outcomes may be impacted by thyroid disorders. Iodine deficiency is also closely linked to a higher risk of miscarriage in this regard. Those who have poorly controlled insulin-dependent diabetes mellitus are at an elevated risk of miscarriage. Miscarriage risk is the same for women with and without diabetes who have their blood sugar under control.

Food poisoning

There is a higher chance of miscarriage if you consume food that has been tainted with listeriosis, toxoplasmosis, or salmonella.

Chorionic villus sampling and amniocentesis

Procedures used to evaluate the fetus include amniocentesis and chorionic villus sampling (CVS). By inserting a needle through the abdomen and into the uterus, a sample of amniotic fluid is taken. Similar steps are used in chorionic villus sampling, except that tissue is sampled instead of fluid. In the first trimester, these procedures are linked to miscarriages and birth abnormalities but not pregnancy loss during the second trimester. About 1% of pregnancies end in miscarriage as a result of invasive prenatal diagnostics, such as chorionic villus sampling (CVS) and amniocentesis.

Surgery

Even the consequences of bariatric surgery are not fully understood when it comes to how they affect pregnancy.

Miscarriage is not increased by pelvic or abdominal surgery. Removal of ovarian cysts and tumors has not been demonstrated to enhance the chance of miscarriage. The excision of the ovary's corpus luteum is an exception to this rule. The pregnancy-maintaining hormones may fluctuate as a result of this.

Medications

The use of antidepressants and spontaneous abortion is not significantly linked. Discontinuing SSRIs before becoming pregnant is not likely to reduce the chance of miscarriage. When studies of low quality are excluded, the risk of miscarriage for women on any antidepressant appears to be statistically less significant.
Medications that raise the chance of miscarriage include:
• Retinoids,
• nonsteroidal anti-inflammatory medications (NSAIDs), such as ibuprofen,
• misoprostol,
• methotrexate,
• Statins

Immunizations

There is no evidence that vaccinations can result in miscarriage. Live vaccines, such as the MMR shot, have the potential to harm developing fetuses because they can pass through the placenta and raise the chance of miscarriage. Therefore, the Centers for Disease Control (CDC) advises against giving live vaccines to pregnant women. There is, however, no conclusive proof that live vaccines raise the risk of miscarriage or fetal defects. MMR, varicella, several strains of the influenza vaccine and rotavirus are a few live vaccines.

Cancer treatments

High doses of ionizing radiation administered to a woman during cancer treatment result in miscarriage. Furthermore, exposure can affect fertility. The risk of future miscarriages rises with the use of chemotherapy medicines for the treatment of pediatric cancer.

History of illnesses

Pre-existing illnesses during pregnancy, including diabetes, polycystic ovarian syndrome (PCOS), hypothyroidism, some viral diseases, and autoimmune disorders, may raise the risk of miscarriage. The chance of miscarriage may rise with PCOS. There have been concerns raised about the validity of two studies that claimed metformin treatment dramatically reduced the likelihood of miscarriage in women with PCOS.] It has not been demonstrated that metformin therapy during pregnancy is safe. The drug's usage to prevent miscarriage was likewise discouraged by the Royal College of Obstetricians and Gynecologists in 2007. The likelihood of miscarriage associated with thrombophilias or other coagulation and bleeding disorders has now been called into question. A miscarriage is more likely in severe hypothyroidism patients. There is no data on how milder hypothyroidism affects the rate of miscarriage. Failure of the uterine lining to adequately prepare for pregnancy is a disorder known as luteal phase deficit (LPD). This may prevent an implanted fertilized egg from doing so or lead to miscarriage.

Preterm birth and miscarriage risk are both raised by Mycoplasma genitalium infection.

The following illnesses can raise the chance of miscarriage: rubella (German measles), CMV, bacterial vaginosis, HIV, chlamydia, gonorrhea, syphilis, and malaria.

State of immunity

Recurrent or late-term miscarriages could have an autoimmune component. A woman's body assaults the developing fetus or obstructs normal pregnancy development in an autoimmune-induced miscarriage. A malformed embryo may result from an autoimmune condition, which increases the risk of miscarriage. As an illustration, Celiac illness has an odds ratio of about 1.4 which increases the risk of miscarriage. Antiphospholipid antibody syndrome can develop as a result of a disruption in regular immunological activity. Whether a woman miscarries repeatedly, she can be examined to see if she has this condition, which will impact her capacity to carry the baby to term. Immunologic variables are involved in about 15% of recurrent miscarriages. Increased risk is linked to the presence of anti-thyroid autoantibodies, with an odds ratio of 3.73 and a 95% confidence interval of 1.8-7.6. Miscarriage risk is also increased by having lupus. Studies using immunohistochemistry on the decidual basalis and chorionic villi revealed a possible link between repeated miscarriages and an immune milieu that is out of balance.

Trauma and Anatomical defects
15% of women who have had three or more recurrent miscarriages have an anatomical abnormality that prevents the pregnancy from being carried to term. The capacity to carry a kid to term is influenced by the uterus' anatomy. Anatomical variations are frequent and occasionally congenital.
Cervical incompetence, also known as cervical insufficiency, affects some women when the cervix cannot remain closed for the whole pregnancy. It does not result in miscarriages during the first trimester. It is linked to an elevated risk of miscarriage in the second trimester. At around 16 to 18 weeks into the pregnancy, it is discovered that premature birth has taken place. Major trauma during the second trimester can cause a

miscarriage.

Smoking

The risk of miscarriage is higher for cigarette and tobacco users. Even though the risk is higher when the pregnant mother smokes, it is elevated regardless of which parent smokes.

The morning sickness

Lower risk is linked to pregnancy-related nausea, vomiting, or morning sickness (NVP). There is currently no consensus about the causes of morning sickness, despite several theories. According to this concept, a lower miscarriage rate would be an expected result of the various food choices made by women experiencing NVP. NVP may act as a defensive mechanism that prevents the mother from consuming foods that are detrimental to the fetus.

Chemicals and Occupational exposure

There may be a correlation between chemical and occupational exposures and pregnancy outcomes. It is nearly never possible to establish a cause-and-effect link. DDT, lead, formaldehyde, arsenic, benzene, and ethylene oxide are the substances that have been linked to an increased incidence of miscarriage. Ultrasound and video display terminals have not been proven to have an impact on miscarriage rates. There is a higher risk of miscarriage in dental practices that employ nitrous oxide without anesthetic gas scavenging equipment. There is a slight increase in the chance of miscarriage for women who use cytotoxic antineoplastic chemotherapy drugs. There is no evidence of a higher risk for cosmetologists.

Other

Miscarriage risk is increased by alcohol consumption. The likelihood of miscarriage rises with cocaine use. Miscarriage has been linked to several infections. These include group B streptococci, Mycoplasma hominis, ureaplasma urealyticum, HIV-1, and syphilis. There is no evidence linking Chlamydia trachomatis, Campylobacter fetus, or Toxoplasma gondii infections to miscarriage. Compared to women with treated chronic endometritis or no chronic endometritis, subclinical infections of the uterine lining, also known as chronic endometritis, are linked to poor pregnancy outcomes.

DIAGNOSIS

Transvaginal ultrasonography is done when there has been blood loss, discomfort, or both. Blood tests (serial HCG tests) can be done to rule out ectopic pregnancy, a potentially fatal condition if a viable intrauterine pregnancy cannot be detected using ultrasonography. Excluding an ectopic pregnancy is crucial if symptoms including anemia, tachycardia, and hypotension are found.

An obstetric ultrasound and a tissue analysis of the expelled material can both confirm a miscarriage. One looks for the results of conception when searching for microscopic pathological symptoms. These can be seen under a microscope and include endometrial background gestational alterations as well as villi, trophoblast, and fetal components. Genetic testing of both parents may be conducted if chromosomal abnormalities are discovered in more than one miscarriage.

MISCARRIAGE CLASSIFICATION

Any bleeding during the early part of pregnancy is a hazard of miscarriage. An investigation may reveal that the fetus is still alive and that the pregnancy is proceeding normally.

An anembryonic pregnancy, often known as an "empty sac" or "blighted ovum," occurs when the gestational sac develops correctly but the embryonic portion of the pregnancy is either absent or the embryonic portion of the pregnancy stops growing extremely early. Approximately 50% of miscarriages are caused by this. All other pregnancies that end in miscarriages are categorized as embryonic miscarriages because an embryo is still present in the gestational sac. Aneuploidy occurs in half of the embryonic miscarriages (an abnormal number of chromosomes). When the cervix has already dilated but the fetus has not yet been released, a miscarriage is unavoidable. This frequently leads to a full miscarriage. There might or might not be heart activity in the fetus.

A complete miscarriage occurs when all fetuses, placentas, amniotic fluid, and membranes have been ejected. These may include the trophoblast, chorionic villi, gestational sac, yolk sac, and fetal pole (embryo).

However, the criterion of pregnancy of uncertain location is satisfied by the presence of a pregnancy test that is still positive and an empty uterus on transvaginal ultrasound. Therefore, it could be necessary to perform follow-up pregnancy tests to make sure that there isn't any residual pregnancy, including ectopic pregnancy.

When only a portion of the fetus leaves the uterus after conception, this is known as an incomplete miscarriage. However, an enlarged endometrial thickness and/or polyp may also be the cause of an increased gap between the uterine walls on transvaginal ultrasonography. When determining whether there are considerable retained products of conception in the uterine cavity, a Doppler ultrasonography may be more useful. Ectopic pregnancy must be ruled out in cases of doubt utilizing methods such as repeated beta-hCG readings.

When the embryo or baby has died but the miscarriage has not yet happened, it is known as a missed miscarriage. Other names for it include missed abortion, quiet miscarriage, and delayed miscarriage. When tissue from a missing or incomplete miscarriage becomes contaminated, it is called a "septic miscarriage," which carries the danger of spreading infection (septicemia), which can be fatal.

Multiple consecutive miscarriages are referred to as recurrent miscarriage (also known as "recurrent pregnancy loss," "recurrent spontaneous abortion," or "habitual abortion"); the precise number used to diagnose this condition varies, but two consecutive miscarriages must occur to meet the requirements.

The likelihood of two consecutive miscarriages is 2.25%, and the likelihood of three consecutive losses is 0.34% if the percentage of pregnancies that end in miscarriage is 15% and miscarriages are assumed to be separate events. Recurrent pregnancies lost are lost 1% of the time. Most women who have experienced two miscarriages (85%) will eventually become pregnant and carry their babies normally.

Depending on how far along in the pregnancy you are, a miscarriage can have a variety of physical symptoms, but for the most part, it hurts or cramps. With lengthier gestations, the size of blood clots and the passed-through pregnancy tissue grows. There is a larger chance of placenta retention after 13 weeks of pregnancy.

ACTIONS TO RESIST MISCARRIAGE

A miscarriage can occasionally be avoided by reducing risk factors. This can involve receiving quality prenatal care, abstaining from drugs and alcohol, avoiding infectious infections, and avoiding x-rays. Finding the miscarriage's underlying cause, particularly in cases of recurrent miscarriage, may assist prevent other pregnancy losses. A person can frequently only take so many steps to stop a miscarriage. Vitamin supplements have not been demonstrated to reduce the risk of miscarriage before or during pregnancy. Women with 1) vaginal bleeding early in their present pregnancy and 2) a prior history of miscarriage have been proven to benefit from progesterone in preventing miscarriage.

Non-modifiable risk factors

Assessments of the following could help prevent miscarriages in future pregnancies:
• Immune health,
• chemical and industrial exposures,
• anatomical flaws,
• Pre-existing or acquired disease during pregnancy,
• polycystic ovarian syndrome,
• prior radiation and chemotherapy exposure,

- medications,
- past surgical procedures,
- endocrine disorders,
- genetic anomalies.

Modifiable risk elements

The risk of miscarriage can be lowered by maintaining a healthy weight and receiving quality prenatal care.
The following can be avoided to reduce some risk factors:
- Smoking
- cocaine usage,
- alcohol consumption,
- malnutrition,
- exposure to substances that can cause miscarriage at work,
- miscarriage-related medications,
- drug abuse.

CHAPTER 5
MANAGEMENT OF MISCARRIAGE

Early miscarriage victims typically don't need any further medical care, although they can still benefit from support and therapy. Most early miscarriages will end on their own, however, in some circumstances, pharmacological treatment or aspiration of the products of conception can be utilized to remove any remaining tissue. Although bed rest has been recommended to avoid miscarriage, this is not helpful. The use of precise medical jargon is advantageous to those who are now experiencing or have just undergone a miscarriage. The skill of the physician to explain concepts in plain language without implying that the lady or the couple is at fault can frequently be used to treat significant discomfort.

Uncertainty exists over the evidence for Rho(D) immune globulin following a spontaneous miscarriage. In the UK, Rho(D) immune globulin is advised for Rh-negative women who need surgery or medication to end the pregnancy after 12 weeks of pregnancy and before 12 weeks of pregnancy.

METHODS

If a total miscarriage is a diagnosis, no treatment is required (so long as ectopic pregnancy is ruled out). There are three possible treatments for incomplete miscarriages, empty sacs, and missed abortions: cautious waiting, medicinal management, and surgical therapy. Most miscarriages (65-80%) will end naturally within two to six weeks if no therapy is given (watchful waiting). The chance of minor bleeding, the need for unplanned surgical treatment, and incomplete miscarriage are higher with this treatment but it avoids the potential side effects and risks of drugs and surgery. Misoprostol (a prostaglandin), either by itself or in conjunction with mifepristone pre-treatment, is typically used as a form of medical treatment.

The uterus is assisted by these drugs in contracting and ejecting the leftover tissue. 95 percent of the time, this works within a few days. It is possible to use a vacuum aspiration or sharp curettage, with vacuum aspiration being the less dangerous and more popular option.

A miscarriage that is both delayed and incomplete.
Treatment for miscarriages that are delayed or incomplete
is based on how much uterine tissue is still present. The
tissue can be surgically removed using vacuum aspiration
or misoprostol as part of the treatment. Studies examining
the anesthetic techniques for surgical management of
incomplete miscarriage have not demonstrated any
advantages to departing from standard practice.

Induced miscarriage

For women who are unable to carry the pregnancy to
term, a skilled healthcare professional may conduct an
induced abortion. Self-induced abortions carried out by
women or non-medical personnel can be risky and are
still a factor in maternal mortality in some nations. It may
be outlawed or subject to severe social stigma in some
places. However, many women in the US opt to safely
induce or manage their abortions.

Sex

To reduce the risk of infection, some organizations advise avoiding intercourse after a miscarriage until the bleeding has stopped. The widespread use of antibiotics to try to prevent infection in partial abortions, however, lacks solid proof. Others advise delaying pregnancy efforts until after the first period to make it simpler to predict the timing of a subsequent pregnancy. No proof getting pregnant during the first cycle has an impact, and subsequent pregnancies that are delivered early may even have a positive impact.

Support

Some organizations offer guidance and information to people who have miscarried. A memorial or burial service is frequently conducted by family and friends. Hospitals can aid in the event's memorialization and offer support. Depending on the location, some people want a private ceremony. As part of the evaluation and treatment process, appropriate assistance is provided along with frequent communication and compassionate counseling. Emotional assistance can be given to people who miscarry suddenly.

Miscarriage Leave

A leave of absence related to a miscarriage is known as a miscarriage leave. The following nations give women who have miscarried compensated or unpaid leave.

• The Philippines offers women who miscarry before 20 weeks of pregnancy or need to have an emergency abortion 60 days of fully paid leave (on the 20th week or after). Up to the fourth pregnancy, the mother's husband is entitled to a seven-day, fully compensated leave.

• Mauritius - two weeks' leave;

• Indonesia - six weeks' leave;

• India - six weeks' leave;

• New Zealand - three days' bereavement leave for both parents;

• Taiwan - five days, one week, or four weeks, depending on how far along the pregnancy was.

OUTCOMES

Emotional and Psychological Effects

Every woman's own miscarriage experience is unique, and women who experience multiple miscarriages may have different reactions to each one.

Since the 1980s, medical professionals have assumed that

having a miscarriage "is a severe loss for all pregnant women" in Western nations. Anxiety, melancholy, or stress might ensue for people involved in a miscarriage. It might affect every member of the family. A grieving process is experienced by a lot of people who have miscarriages. It is common to experience "prenatal attachment," which can be interpreted as parental sensitivity, love, and preoccupation with the unborn child. Immediately following a miscarriage is typically when serious emotional effects are felt. The loss experienced by some when an ectopic pregnancy is ended is possible. The reality of the loss can take weeks for some people. It can be difficult to offer family support to families who have lost a child because some people find solace in talking about miscarriages while others may find it hard to do so. The father could experience a similar sense of loss. Sometimes it can be more difficult for males to express their sentiments of loss and grief. After a few weeks have passed since the miscarriage, some women can start making plans for their subsequent pregnancies. Planning a second pregnancy can be challenging for some people. The loss is acknowledged by certain facilities. Infants can be named and held by their parents. Mementos like images and footprints are possible to give them. A memorial or funeral service may be held by some. Planting a tree could be one way they show their sadness. Delaying sexual activity after a miscarriage is advised by several health organizations. After about three to four months, the menstrual cycle should return. The treatment they received from doctors and nurses reportedly left women feeling unsatisfied.

Subsequent pregnancies

After a miscarriage, some parents want to start trying for a baby right away. Deciding to attempt another pregnancy can be challenging. Some factors could make parents want to try again. There might be a feeling of urgency for older mothers. Other parents are confident that future pregnancies will probably be successful. Many people are wary and want to know the likelihood of having second or more miscarriages. Before attempting another pregnancy, several medical professionals advise the women to have one menstrual cycle. This is due to the potential difficulty in determining the date of conception. Additionally, the first menstrual period following a miscarriage may be significantly longer or shorter than anticipated. Parents who have had a late miscarriage, a molar pregnancy, or who are undergoing tests may be advised to wait even longer. Depending on advice from their doctor, some parents decide to wait six months.

The likelihood of suffering another miscarriage varies depending on the cause. After a molar pregnancy, the likelihood of experiencing another miscarriage is extremely low. After the third miscarriage, the likelihood of having another one increases. In some places, pre-conception care is offered.

Future Cardiovascular Disease
Miscarriage significantly increases the risk of developing coronary artery disease later in life, but not the cerebrovascular illness.

CHAPTER 6
SIGNS AND SYMPTOMS OF PREGNANCY

1. Amenorrhea (stopped menstrual flow) (ceased menstrual flow)

The absence of a menstrual period in a woman of reproductive age is known as amenorrhea. Most frequently, physiological amenorrhea is encountered during pregnancy and lactation (breastfeeding). Menstruation is absent throughout childhood and following menopause, which is not the reproductive years.

Amenorrhea is a symptom that could have a wide range of reasons. Primary amenorrhea is characterized by either normal secondary sexual characteristics without menarche by age 15 or the absence of secondary sexual characteristics by age 13 with no menarche.

Developmental issues such as the congenital lack of the uterus, the inability of the ovary to produce or preserve egg cells, or a delay in pubertal development could be the root of the problem. The absence of menses for three months in a woman with previously regular menstruation, or six months in the case of women with a history of oligomenorrhoea, is referred to as secondary amenorrhoea, the cessation of menstrual cycles following menarche. It is frequently brought on by hormonal imbalances from the pituitary and hypothalamus glands, early menopause, intrauterine scarring, or eating problems.

Classification

Amenorrhea can be primary or secondary.

Primary Amenorrhea: Primary amenorrhoea is the lack of menstruation in a woman by the age of 16. Females who have not attained menarche by the age of 14 and who show no symptoms of secondary sexual characteristics (thelarche or pubarche) are also regarded as having primary amenorrhea. The constitutional delay of puberty, Turner syndrome, and Mayer-Rokitansky-Küster-Hauser

(MRKH) syndrome are a few examples of amenorrhea.

Secondary Amenorrhea: Secondary amenorrhoea is the absence of menstruation for three months in a woman with a history of regular cyclic bleeding or six months in a woman with a history of irregular menstrual cycles. Hypothyroidism, hyperthyroidism, hyperprolactinemia, polycystic ovarian syndrome, primary ovarian insufficiency, and functional hypothalamic amenorrhea are some examples of secondary amenorrhea.

2. Tender, swollen breasts: Hormonal changes early in pregnancy may make your breasts sensitive and painful. After a few weeks, the uneasiness should lessen as your body gets used to the hormonal fluctuations.

3. Vomiting or feeling queasy: One to two months after becoming pregnant, morning sickness, which can strike at any time of the day or night, frequently begins. Although some women experience nausea more frequently than others, some never do. Hormones associated with pregnancy most likely have a role in morning sickness, even though the precise cause is uncertain.

4. Light spotting: One of the earliest signs of pregnancy could be this symptom. When the fertilized egg attaches to the lining of the uterus, this process is known as implantation bleeding and takes place 10 to 14 days following fertilization. Usually, the time that you would expect to get your period coincides with the onset of implantation bleeding. Females do not, however, all have it.

5. More frequent urination: You might find that you urinate more frequently than usual. Your body makes more blood when you're pregnant, which leads your kidneys to process extra fluid, which then builds up in your bladder.

6. Fatigue: Excessive fatigue is one of the most noticeable early pregnancy symptoms. In the first trimester of pregnancy, it is uncertain who or what specifically causes drowsiness. But fatigue might be influenced by a substantial rise in progesterone levels in the first trimester of pregnancy.

7. Headache: Early in pregnancy, headaches are typical.

They are typically brought on by elevated blood volume and changed hormone levels. If your headaches don't go away or if they're particularly painful, call your doctor.

8. Spotting: In the first trimester of pregnancy, some women may suffer minor bleeding and spotting. The most frequent cause of this bleeding is implantation. Typically, one to two weeks after fertilization, implants take place. Additionally, relatively simple issues like an infection or irritation might cause early pregnancy bleeding. The latter frequently affects the cervix's surface (which is very sensitive during pregnancy).
A major pregnancy issue, such as a miscarriage, an ectopic pregnancy, or a placenta previa, can occasionally be detected by bleeding. In case you have any worries, always call your doctor.

9. Weight gain: During the first few months of pregnancy, you can anticipate gaining between 1 and 4 pounds. In your second trimester, weight gain starts to become more obvious.

10. Hypertension brought on by pregnancy: Sometimes during pregnancy, high blood pressure, or hypertension, develops. Your risk may be increased by several things,

such as:
• being obese or overweight
• smoking
• a history of pregnancy-induced hypertension or a family
history of it

11. Heartburn: Pregnancy hormones may occasionally
cause the valve between your stomach and esophagus to
loosen. Heartburn can occur when stomach acid spills out.

12. Constipation: Early pregnancy hormone changes can
cause your digestive system to slow down. As a result,
constipation might set in.

13. Cramps: You can experience a pulling sensation
similar to menstruation cramps when the muscles in your
uterus start to stretch and expand. Along with your
cramps, spotting or blood may indicate a miscarriage or
an ectopic pregnancy.

14. Back discomfort: In the early stages of pregnancy,
hormones, and muscle stress are the main causes of back
pain. Later, your back pain can become worse due to your
increased weight and an altered center of gravity. About

half of all expectant mothers, report experiencing back pain.

15. Anemia: Pregnant women are more likely to develop anemia, which can result in symptoms including dizziness and lightheadedness.
Low birth weight and early birth can result from the disease. Anemia is typically screened for during prenatal care.

16. Depression: Pregnant women experience depression between 14 and 23% of the time. Your numerous biological and mental changes could be significant factors. If you don't feel like yourself, be sure to tell your doctor.

17. Insomnia: Another typical early pregnancy symptom is insomnia. Hormonal fluctuations, physical discomfort, and stress can all be contributing factors. You can improve your sleep quality with a balanced diet, sound sleeping practices, and yoga stretches.

18. Breast changes: One of the first telltale indicators of pregnancy is a change in the breasts. Your breasts may start to feel sensitive, swollen, and generally heavy or full before you're far enough along for a positive test. Additionally, the areolae may darken and your nipples may enlarge and become more sensitive.

19. Acne: Many women have acne in the first trimester of pregnancy as a result of elevated androgen levels. Your skin may become more oily due to these hormones, which may clog pores. Acne during pregnancy typically subsides after the baby is born.

20. Hip pain: Hip pain is a frequent pregnancy symptom that tends to get worse as the pregnancy progresses. There are numerous potential causes, such as:
• alterations in posture;
• sciatica;
• pressure on your ligaments;
• a bigger uterus

21. Diarrhea: During pregnancy, it's common to experience diarrhea as well as other digestive issues. Possible causes include adjustments in hormone levels, dietary changes, and increased stress. Make an appointment with your doctor if diarrhea persists for more than a few days to prevent dehydration.

CHAPTER 7

12 EFFECTIVE STRATEGIES TO PREVENT TEEN PREGNANCY

1. Sexuality Education

Teenagers might not have received sexual education or know how to avoid unintended pregnancies and STDs (STDs). Due to peer pressure, they might also engage in unprotected sexual behavior.

How to assist:

• Teach teenagers about sexuality.

• Encourage youth development initiatives that encourage open discussion about sexuality among adolescents.

• Inform them about issues including contraception, STDs, and HIV.

• Bring communities and families together to discuss sexuality issues without encountering any sociocultural barriers.

• Discuss the dangers of unprotected sex and teenage pregnancies on one's health.

Brief fact

Teenagers can acquire the skills they need to grow up to be kind and sympathetic adults by participating in sex education that is inclusive and culturally appropriate.

2. **Use more contraceptives.**

Adopting effective contraceptive methods (condoms, hormonal, and emergency contraceptives) can help avoid teenage pregnancies, according to WHO studies carried out in China, India, Kenya, Thailand, and other nations. However, the majority of teenagers are either unable to purchase contraceptives or are not knowledgeable about how to use them.

How to help:

• Shed societal stigma and inform youngsters about contraception.

• The American Academy of Family Physicians, the American Academy of Pediatrics, and the American Medical Association advise doctors and healthcare professionals to provide advice about contraceptives and sexual activity.

3. Lessen the use of forced sex

According to studies carried out in nations like Botswana, Kenya, and India, gender norms can lead to coerced sex of females.
How to help:
• Give females confidence by providing them with support and security.
• Develop sensible plans for enhancing social networks, educating people about life skills, and fostering self-esteem.
• Work to alter social attitudes and social norms that are currently in place around forced sex and sexual violence.

4. Prevent young marriage

In developing nations like Afghanistan, India, Kenya, and Nepal, the proportion of girls who marry before the age of 15 is around 14%. Early marriage causes early pregnancies and has bad effects on reproductive health. In addition to facing poverty and inadequate education, young brides also jeopardize the future of their families.

How to aid:

• Encourage girls to attend education to reduce the likelihood of early marriage. Their improved family care and beneficial social influence are both facilitated by education.

• Motivate teens to remain attention-focused and avoid distractions while pursuing their career ambitions.

5. **Pay attention to media influence**

In the US, sexual conduct is highlighted in one out of every three television shows. According to research, watching television episodes that portray sexual conduct in young people leads to their involvement in non-marital sexual activity.

Helping ways:

• Keep an eye on the media that kids read, listen to, or watch.

• Disputing what they are learning from these programs.

• Because low-risk sexual behaviors are encouraged through widespread media campaigns in industrialized nations like France, the Netherlands, and Germany, teen pregnancies are significantly lower than they are in the US.

6. **Offer advice to male teenagers**

Male teenagers have more partners and engage in sexual activity earlier than female teenagers, but they show fewer signs of reproductive anxiety. Girls are the primary target of the majority of health clinics and teen pregnancy prevention initiatives.

• By focusing educational initiatives on both boys and girls, teen pregnancy can be effectively addressed.

• Educate male teenagers on STIs, risky conduct, and sexually transmitted infections.

• Promote the use of condoms among teenage boys to ward against illnesses and pregnancy. Inform them of postcoital and alternative forms of contraception.

• Assist young men in understanding what it means to be a partner.

7. **Offer career advice**

Because of their difficult financial situation, many females married young. Therefore, programs that emphasize job advice can persuade individuals to pursue education and provide for their families rather than get married young.

How to help:

• Educate young women from less affluent families on their options for jobs and higher education.

• In 80 villages in India (near Delhi), recruiters sponsored three annual workshops for young women to tell them about employment options and techniques for applying for jobs. These seminars assisted 76 to 81% of the women in delaying marriage and childbirth by enrolling in diploma programs.

8. Education about abstinence

Abstinence is the decision to refrain from sexual activity to reduce the risk of becoming pregnant. Most teenagers choose to put off having sex until they are older. Youths must follow this responsible choice without being swayed by peer pressure.

How to help:

• Help kids select friends and partners who accept their decision to abstain from drugs and alcohol;
• Encourage youth to avoid substance misuse;
• The Michigan Abstinence Program encourages teens to refrain from sexual activity and other harmful behaviors including using drugs, alcohol, or tobacco to improve their overall health.

9. Insurance for contraception

Because they cannot afford them, teenagers might not use contraceptive techniques. Contraception is not typically covered by private insurance plans.

How to help:
• Teen pregnancy rates are significantly lower in the Netherlands, Germany, and France, where contraceptive pills and devices are covered by insurance;
• Youth should have easy access to contraception.

10. Encourage gender equality

Gender ideology has an impact on how young men and women act and make decisions about contraception. Social norms hold that young women should avoid disclosing any sexual engagement, whereas young men should do the exact reverse. When it comes to using contraception, the same philosophies are presented. The wishes and opinions of women are frequently suppressed by these gender disparities, which increases the number of teenage pregnancies.

How to Help:

• Change the social norms that produce gender differences.

• To spur a rise in the use of contraceptives, promote gender equality.

• Encourage female empowerment so they can speak up.

11. Establish positive connections with kids

Children might become content and confident if their parents have a nice relationship. They'll be conscious of their obligations and moral principles.

• Pay attention to the information your kids share.

• Show them respect, courtesy, and kindness.

• Encourage your kids' endeavors and be proud of them.

• Encouragement to improve one's confidence and

self-worth.

12. Keep an eye on activities

Find out if your children are safe and what they spend the majority of their time doing. You must keep a tight eye on their behavior as a parent.

How to help:

• Get to know the friends and family of the kids.

• Find out the ideals that their friends uphold by routinely speaking with them.

• Keep up with your kids' activities.

• If you discover anything worrisome, express your concern right away.

Quick Advice

Limit your dating to partners with an age difference of no more than two years, as power imbalances may lead to unprotected or unwelcome sex.

PROGRAMS TO PREVENT TEENAGE PREGNANCIES

Governments all across the world implement various strategies to reduce teenage pregnancy. Effective programs include:

1. Taking Pride in Prevention (TPIP): This Michigan initiative aims to reduce teen pregnancies and STDs by educating and motivating young people to use contraception and abstinence. To lower the teen pregnancy rate, it specifically targets young people between the ages of 12 and 19.

2. Development Initiative Supporting Healthy Adolescents (DISHA): This Indian program educates teenagers on sex education, contraception, money management, future jobs, and life skills in addition to offering health care to individuals.

3. Carrera/Home Children's Society Program: This 1984-founded US initiative offers young people services related to their health, employment, way of life, sexuality, and education. It originally began as an after-school program for kids ages 13 to 15 and older.

4. The Zomba Cash Transfer Program: This Malawi initiative gives females and recent dropouts $10 and their school costs to return to the classroom.